A Bear's
Sleepy Journey

By
Kate Mullin

Illustration by Liz Mullin

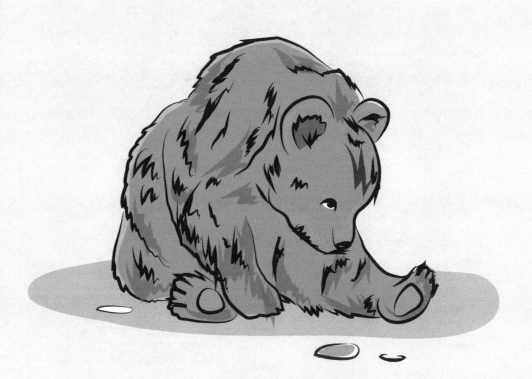

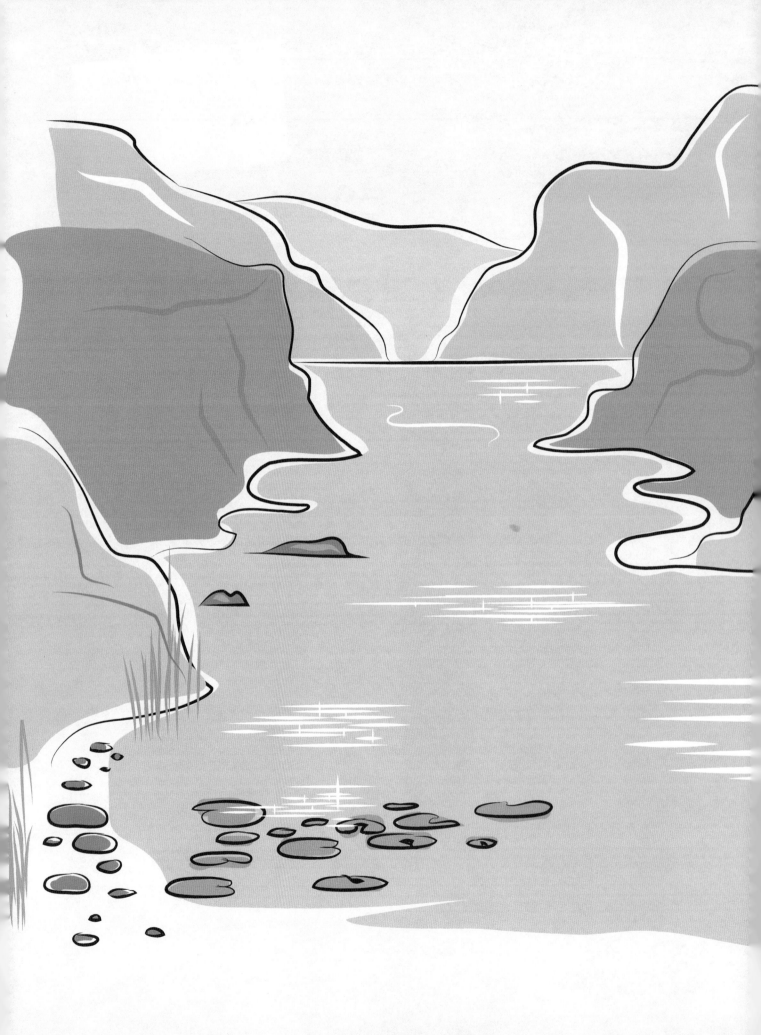

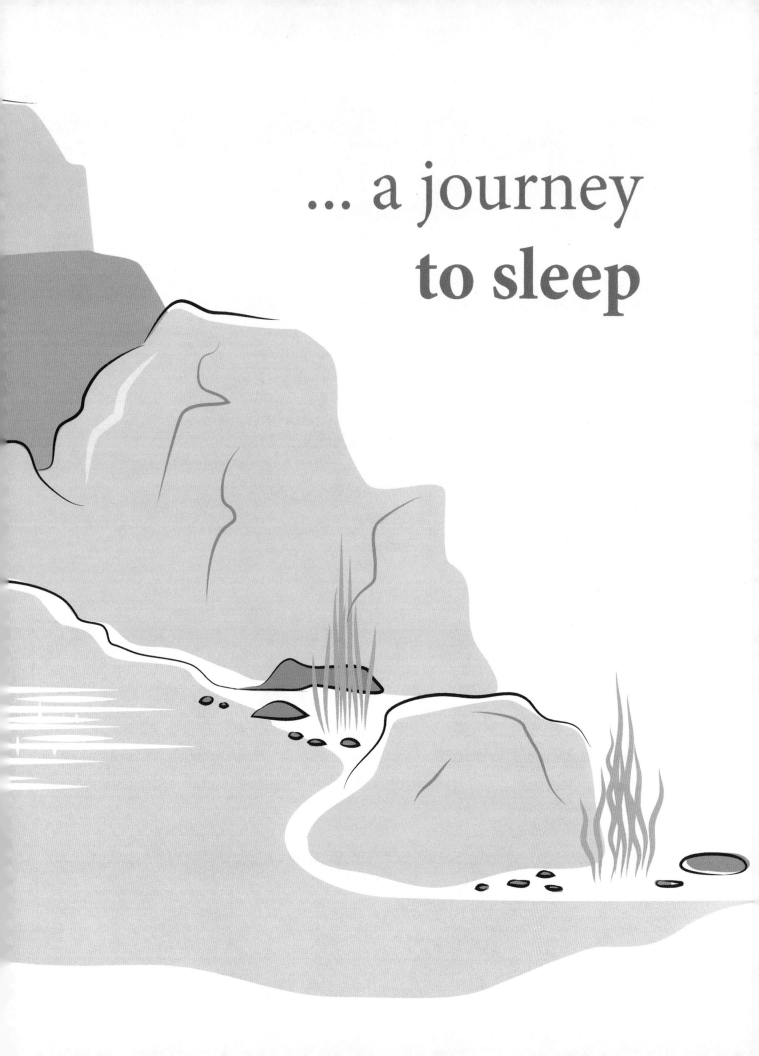

... a journey
to sleep

Acknowledgements

Dedicated to

Eloise, Mae, Austin, Emma and Chase

Special thanks to Philomena Shotton

First Published April 2016

Text © copyright 2016 by Kate Mullin

Illustration © copyright 2016 by Liz Mullin

© A Bear's Sleepy Journey

A Bear's
Sleepy
Journey

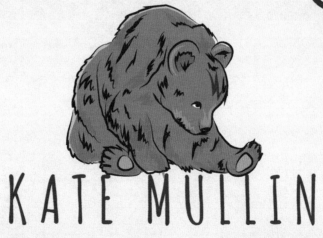

KATE MULLIN

A Bear's Sleepy Journey

Specially designed to help children get to sleep.

Information for the reader.

I have written this book using special language and a psychological approach, so it is a fantastic way of using the subconscious mind to make changes and help your child to fall asleep. It uses my specially designed script with some hypnotic language, story telling metaphors and relaxation techniques which will help your child relax, making bedtime a happy occasion!

I have designed the story for the subconscious mind to respond to the positive commands (see **bold text**) throughout, so that your child will feel safe and relaxed and thus able to fall asleep. Some sentences may seem strange and long-winded but 'bear' with me as this will help your child's subconscious mind switch off and relax deeply. The bold text throughout the book indicates the positive commands. You, the reader can emphasis these parts in clear sleepy voice to help the idea of the story.

Your child should be lying down and comfortable to listen to the story. Check they are not too hot or too cold. They may need to hear it a few times to relax and enjoy it. They can close their eyes when they are ready and use their imagination while listening. All of these techniques should help your child to sleep.

I hope that this book helps your child to sleep with the least amount of effort, and gives you some new tools to use for effective bedtime results for sleep, though of course all children are different and I can make no guarantees and take no responsibility for the outcome.

It's worth mentioning a **warning** about using the book carefully as it may cause sleepiness. Do not read the book out loud close to someone driving or in a vehicle or doing any activity that requires them to be awake!

There is also a Sleep Certificate to photocopy or cut out and use as a reward for sleep. This is another way in which you can get the best possible outcome by rewarding the behaviour that you want. You can set the rules for when your child will get their sleep certificate, maybe after three consecutive nights of sleep, or whatever you feel is appropriate for your child.

This is a great way for a bedtime story to be fun and sleepy at the same time.
Happy dreams and success!

Kate

A Bear's Sleepy Journey

I'm wondering if you're comfortable? Are you lying down with your head on the pillow? If the answer is yes, then we can begin our sleepy story. You're going to travel to a special place with Drowsy bear to The Rainbow Caves where all the secrets of **sleep can be found**. Drowsy bear is very special just like you. He doesn't find it **easy to go to sleep quickly every night**. I'm wondering if you can you help him with his sleepy journey?

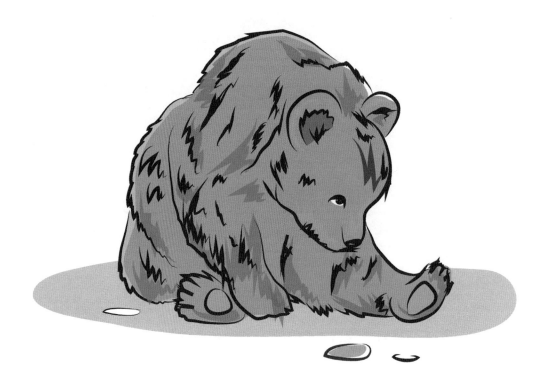

Lie still and **listen to the sound of your heart beat**. You **can close your eyes** at anytime. You can try if you want to not **fall asleep** by making your eyes wider and wider, or you can choose to relax your eyes so gently that they are so relaxed . This is a sleepy story so don't worry if **you find that you fall asleep. You can fall asleep** whenever you want. Listen quietly. Can hear the sound of your breathing? Shhh all is well. Listen... some words **you will hear** and others **will float away,** but **you will hear** the words you need. Your arms and legs might feel floaty as **you listen**, or your arms and legs might feel heavy too, or you can feel happy sleepy tingles as they spread to your fingers and arms... shoulders... relaxing tingles all around your neck... sleepy head and tummy... sleepy chest... sleepy hips... as you float deeper into relaxing every part of you, sleepy knees... sleepy ankles... sleepy toes.

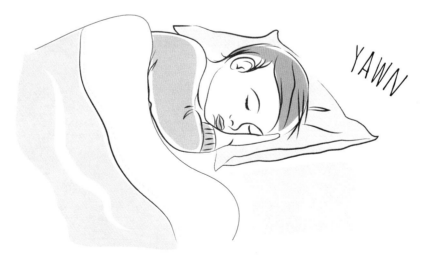

Note to reader - Read slowly when you see the '...' or pause a few moments when reading these relaxing sentences. Yawning will also help your child respond and feel sleepy too.

As you **listen you might feel floaty sleep arrive** at any time and **you can take** it for Drowsy bear. He will be very happy that you can help him sleep. Drowsy bear will be so happy to **know how to sleep every night**. You can **discover the answers to sleep** in The Rainbow Caves for Drowsy bear. Let's drift there now.

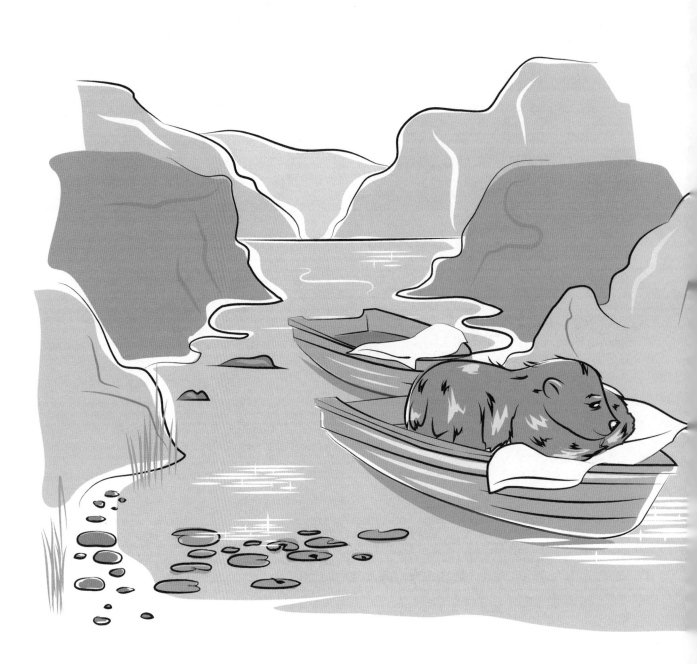

All you have to do is **relax** and snuggle down.

"Let's float to The Rainbow Caves," says Drowsy.

Remember to **close your eyes** as you listen. Use your imagination (a picture in the mind) to see a lovely stream in front of you, with water flowing and there you see lots of tiny special 'pillow boats' inside floating along the stream, like little seats to take you to The Rainbow Caves.

Drowsy is getting smaller now, like a tiny bear as he jumps onto a pillow boat in the water. Can you see him as he starts to float down the stream? You find yourself getting smaller and smaller too. You want to follow him all the way down. You see a boat with a large pillow in it float by. This is your 'pillow boat.' You hop on as it takes **you deeper and deeper down** along the stream, **as you float away, following Drowsy bear.**

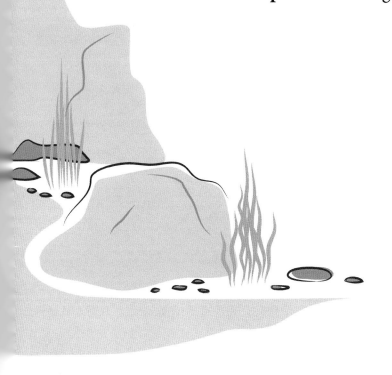

Drowsy is getting carried gently down the stream. You know **you can float down** the stream so easily, like Drowsy bear as you get carried safely on your pillow in your boat. You float through the water and dip your hand in the stream, as the cool water trickles through your fingers. How lovely it feels!

Soon you see the sleepy caves. Drowsy pulls his pillow boat to the waters edge. You stop your pillow boat and **follow Drowsy** to the caves to **find the answers to sleep** here.

You see the first cave in front of you.

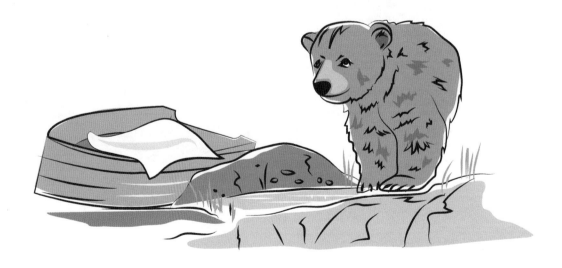

It is a red cave. Everything in here is red. It has a warm red glow. It feels so warm and you can see the red glow in the cave.

"Are you ready to explore and **look for the things we need in the caves**?" said Drowsy **taking a big deep breath. You follow.** The Rainbow Caves will give you lots of **help along the way.**

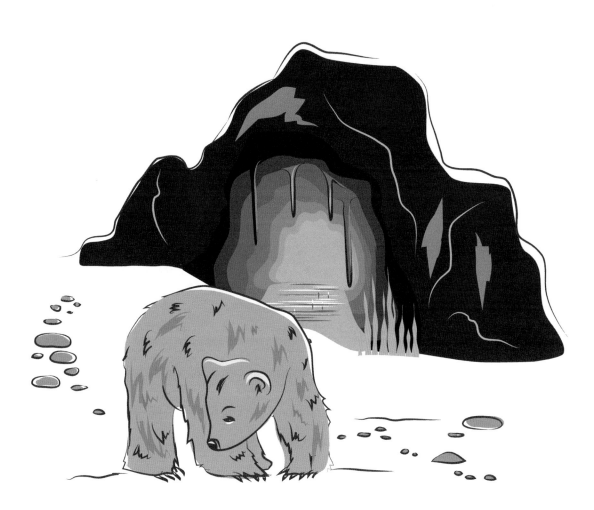

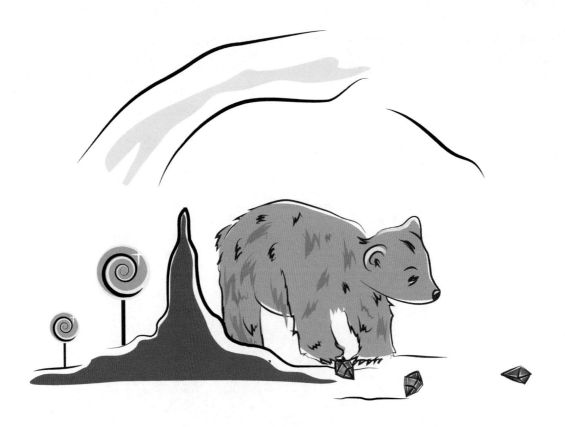

The first cave is red. As you wander with Drowsy into the red cave you **notice how confident you feel**. You know you can help Drowsy **fall asleep now**. You see everything is a warm red and makes you feel toasty and safe, like a log fire at Christmas, or candy canes with swirls of red around each stick. It is lovely in the red cave and as you walk through it, and it glows. **You feel so wonderful and confident.** You can **take the confidence** you feel in here with you at all times. Confidence to **sleep through the night.**

Now in front of you, you see Drowsy is heading to a new cave. It is an orange cave. As you walk into the cave, it has an orange glow. It feels warm and cosy, with warm camp fires glowing. In here you see wonderful orange swirls of warmth and feel it all around you. You warm your hands by the fire and **notice all the strength you feel** in this cave. Drowsy is smiling with a warm glow on his face. You **feel stronger and happier** as you walk through the orange cave. The next cave is yellow.

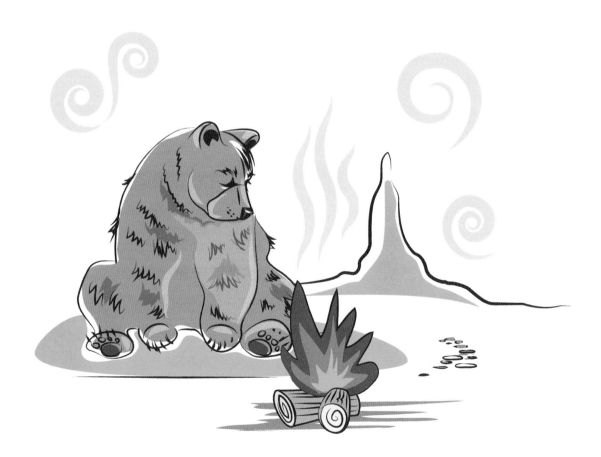

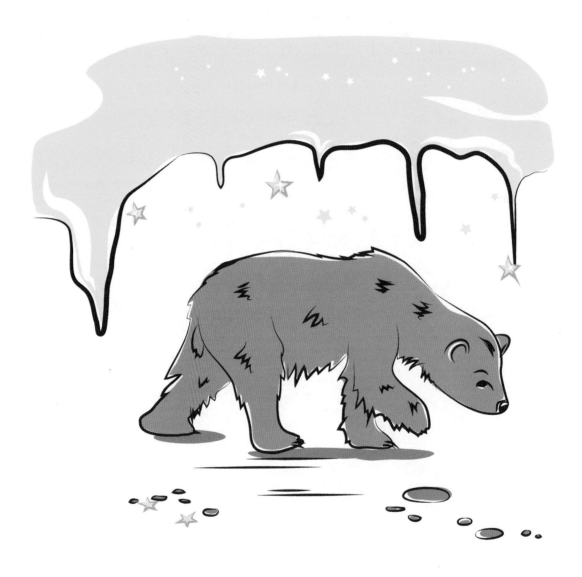

Now in the yellow cave, of course it has a yellow glow. You walk into the cave and it shines so brightly just like you! In here you see special shiny stars all over the walls. You notice each star has a number on it. You go over and take the stars. You notice a special yellow bag appears across your shoulder to put all the stars in. You start counting the numbers. **Number ten, number nine**, you enjoy picking the stars from the cave. You are so busy choosing your numbers that soon they are all gone. Drowsy is picking stars too, **eight, seven,** you find **six and then five** and **number four** and he picks up **number three and number two**, and then you find star **number one** and put it in your special bag. The yellow bag will keep them **safe for you**. The bag **feels a bit heavy** with all those stars, but you know all the numbers are gone, so **you know you have to move forwards** into the next cave.

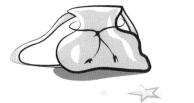
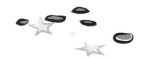

It is a green cave. It has a green glow. Here you see lots of green plants, leaves and shoots. You feel **you can grow** in here like the green plants, you **notice how you can learn** from the plants as they grow **they know exactly what they need**, just as you know when **you need to sleep** and dream. You see a watering can and begin to water the plants and they smile back at you, pleased that **you know what they need**, just as **you know what is good** for the plants. They **know that when you sleep well all night you will feel fresh and ready for the new day ahead** every morning.

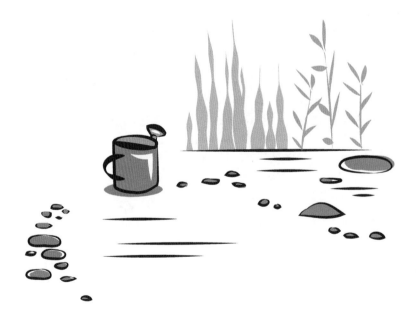

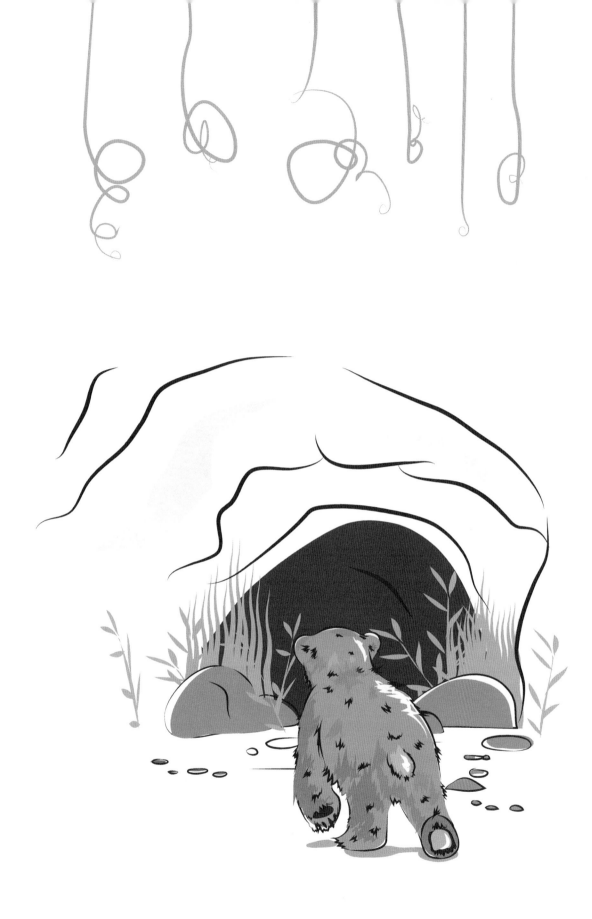

Now up ahead is a blue cave. It had a blue glow. You walk into the blue cave. It has blue pools of water on the ground and blue water drips down from the walls. It is pretty and so calm and peaceful. The blue water drips; **down, down, down,** calmer and clearer with every drop. **You feel peaceful** here. You see Drowsy is enjoying the pools too.

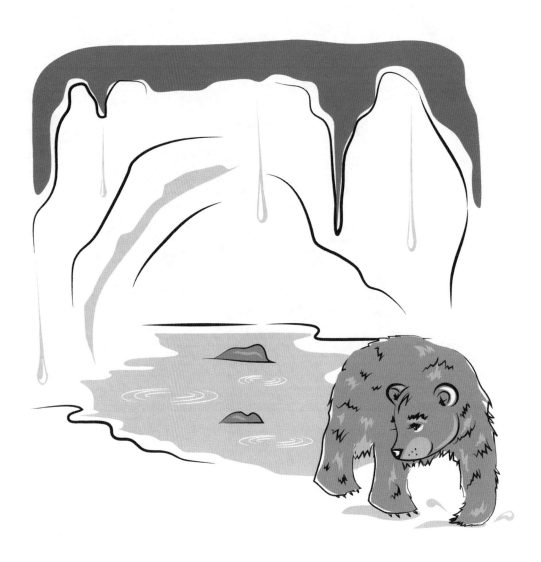

Now up ahead you see the last cave all shiny and silvery white. It has a large white bed with the softest pillows and a fluffy duvet. The bed has a name on it. It is your name. It is written on the bed, can you see it? You climb into your special bed and snuggle down. Next to the bed is a big armchair. The armchair has Drowsy bears name on it and there is a huge story book lying there. Drowsy sits on his special chair and picks up his special storybook. You see the word, 'Sleep' on the book. Drowsy opens it and starts to read, he feels strangely tired. His arms and legs feel heavy. Can you feel it too? The book has a strange gold mist that blows gently onto his face as he reads. As the mist fills the air, Drowsy starts to yawn.

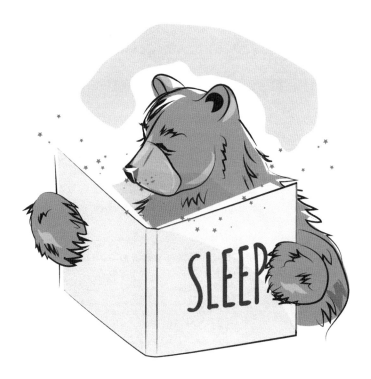

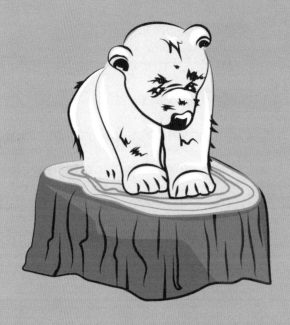

Drowsy reads, "This is the story of Bobo bear. A lively polar bear who loved to play all day long, swimming and fishing. Bobo was an explorer too. He loved adventures and travelling as far as he could. He lived in the North Pole. It is such a beautiful place to live, as you can imagine. He had heard there was a wise old bear who could help **people find their sleepy dreams**. He was the Lord of the Arctic bear, a bear who knows everything about sleep. Bobo wanted to see if he could find him. He told his mum, 'I must find this wise bear and ask him my questions, he will have the answers for me.' His mum said he could go, but he must be back in time for bed, but it was not that **easy to listen to his mum** when he wanted to explore.

He had heard the bear lived across the snowy plains, he knew he could reach the there and be back in time for bed. So Bobo set off to find the wise bear. He set off but it was a stormy day. He walked through a blizzard where the snow flew into his face and it was hard to **keep going**. His feet sank into snowy piles, as he continued to walk onwards to **find the sleepy** bear. He walked for miles. The journey seemed endless at times, but **he was determined** to get to the Lord of the Arctic bear. At times he wanted to **stop and curl up**, to make a snowy den but he knew he had to find the Lord of the Arctic bear.

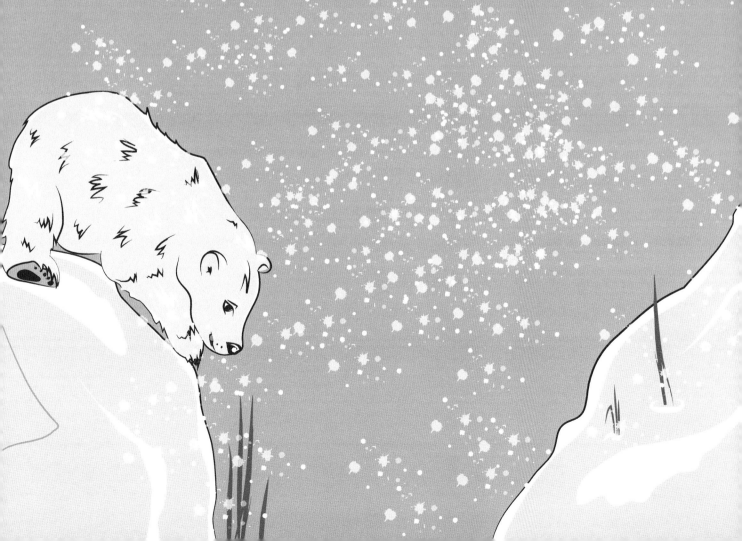

Ahead of him was a frozen lake. He started to walk across it, but as he walked the ice started to melt. He started to **float away down** the lake on a piece of broken ice. He was swept along, further down into a snowy blizzard. It was hard to see what was ahead, as **he tried to keep his eyes open but he had to close them** to keep the snowstorm out. The speed of the ice was moving fast, as **he continued onwards and further down he went**. He clung on but it was no good the ice was moving and he **had to go with it** now.

"Hello?" he called. He could hear his voice travel for miles but nothing came back. He sat for a while wondering what he should do. He closed his eyes to think but **he couldn't think of anything, all his thoughts were gone now.**

A few moments later a seal swam by. It stopped.

"Are you lost?" It asked Drowsy. It yawned. It had been napping.

"Yes, I'm looking for the Lord of the Arctic bear," he said. "Do you know if he lives near here?"

"Yes I know him. You need to **go a little further down** that way and you see the snowy hill. He lives just behind there," said the seal.

He will be asleep in the land of dreams, but he will answer your questions while he sleeps. He is always listening, if you say the right words."

"What should I say?"

"Oh well you simply go over to the bear and lift his ear, then you whisper your question, without waking him, and he will answer you. Just speak from you heart and let the words flow. **Your heart will know what to do**. You must match your question to your heart and **your head will follow**," said the seal.

"Thank you," said Bobo, even though he didn't really know what the seal meant but it did not matter as **he felt much calmer** after talking to her.

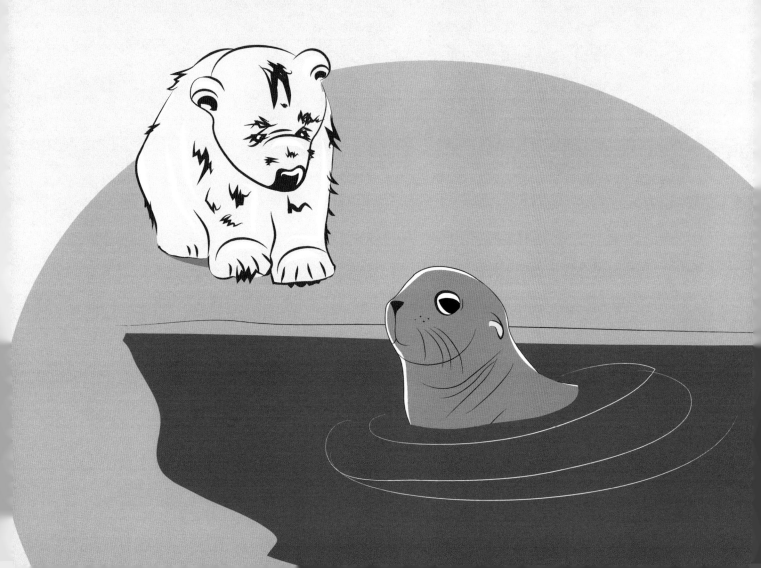

Bobo **followed all the instructions**. He knew the Lord of the Arctic bear had the important secrets of helping bears to dream. He had helped so many bears no matter how big the problem he always solved it, every time. Bobo walked over the snowy hills and knew he was close. Then he saw just ahead of him a clearing and a big cave. Inside the cave was a huge bear. **The big bear was sleeping** just as the seal had told him.

Bobo felt **happy to have found the sleep**ing bear. He crept over as he didn't want to wake him. He knew he should whisper his question and the bear would send him the answers in his sleepy dreams.

Bobo walked over and lifted the bear's ear. He was careful to **be quiet and still** as he did this, so that the bear would **stay asleep**.
He whispered his question and the bear opened his eye slowly and then closed it again. The bear spoke in a low deep voice, "When you want to go to sleep, put all this relaxation into your eyes and relax them as much as you can."

A sparkling golden mist came out of the bear's mouth as he spoke in a deep low voice, the beautiful wisdom flowed from the bear.

Bobo felt strangely confident, he **wanted to go straight home to his bed and dream**. It was just like **he had been filled with dreams**. He set off home to **go to bed and go to sleep as his mummy would expect as it was bed time now**. His little legs carried him all the way home.

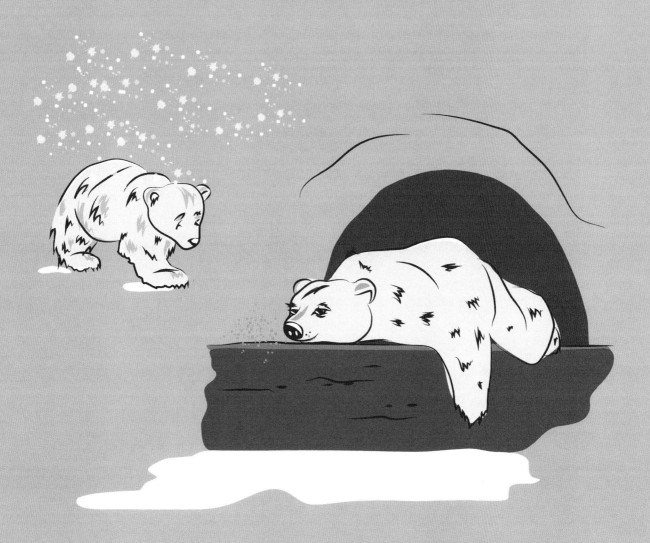

Drowsy bear had finished the story. He stretched and let his body sink into the big comfy chair. He yawned one last yawn and sank back, fast asleep.

We can all sleep and we can all dream, and then in the morning we will wake up refreshed after a really good night's sleep. And again the next night and the night after that, and the night after that **we will find ourselves drifting to sleepy dreams, as easily** as Bobo and Drowsy. We **know it really is simply a case of letting ourselves float away** into our dreams.

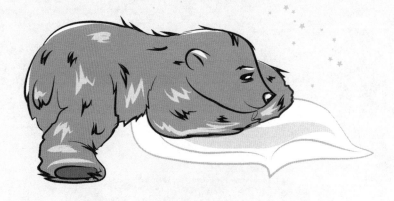

Sleepy bear dreams... Night Night!

Interesting fact for reader!

**Lord of the Arctic is one of the names for large
polar bears given in Norway.**

In the story, it represents the subconscious mind perfectly as a metaphor of the power it has on beliefs and values, so it can program in sleepy behaviour, night after night. This should naturally help your child subconsciously follow a pattern to get to sleep, which becomes a good habit. The subconscious mind will obey the commands and help maintain consistent behaviour, which is also rewarded with a Sleep certificate. This builds in a happy association with getting to sleep night after night.

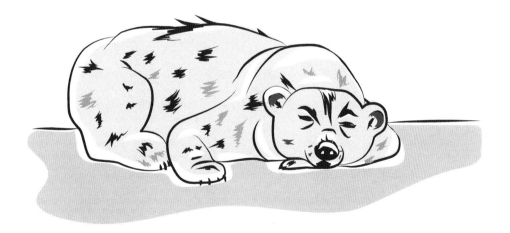

From the Author

I hope you enjoyed reading, 'A Bear's Sleepy Journey' book as much as I enjoyed writing it!

The sleepy bear book is a favourite of mine because I love bears, and it shows how powerful stories can be. I am writing more special stories like this to help children reach their goals. I also think books give parents a great tool to start discussions about the world, when reading with their children. I would love to hear your experiences of using the book and see all those Sleepy Bear Certificates being used. I look forward to hearing all your success stories!

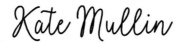

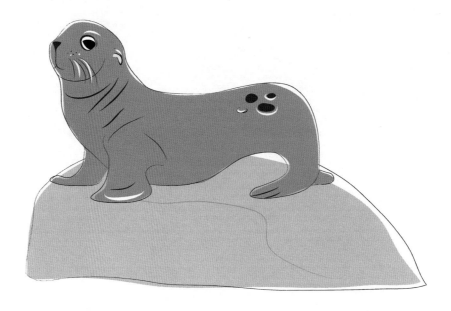

About the Author

Kate's is a teacher, hypnotherapist and NLP practitioner. She has a bachelor's degree in Social Policy BA(Hons) and a PGCE in Education with English. She has taught in schools for over twenty years and still works as a teacher. After gaining a diploma in hypnotherapy and counselling, she has developed these psychological approaches in her writing and with clients. She now enjoys the flexibility of writing, counselling and teaching. She is passionate about creativity and behaviour change in health and education.

This special book was designed with her sister Liz who illustrated the book. Liz has a Psychology and Physiology degree BSc(Hons) and works as an illustrator and digital designer.

Their other books include -
'Pongy Stinkbelly finds a friend' available on Amazon. This story covers themes of self acceptance and empathy. It has been a hit with children, parents and grandparents all over the world!

Sweet dreams

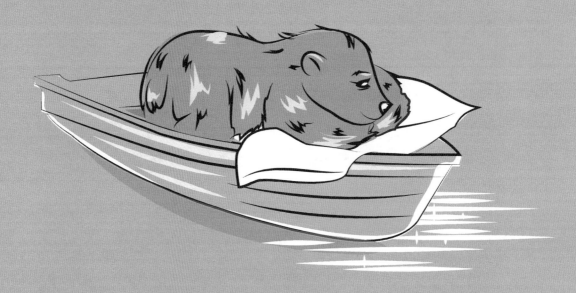

Goodnight!

CERTIFICATE
OF SLEEP

This certificate is awarded to

_____

for excellence at bedtime and sleep success

Date: _____

Given by: **Drowsy Bear**

_____

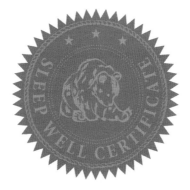

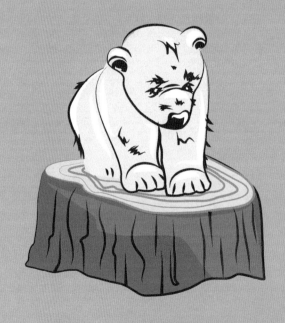